THE GLUCOSE GODDESS BOOK

The Life-Changing Power of Balancing Blood Sugar Effectively

James Cooper

Copyright Page

Copyright © 2023 [James Cooper]

Reservation of rights. With the exception of brief quotations incorporated into critical reviews and certain other noncommercial uses allowed by copyright law, no part of this publication may be reproduced, distributed, or transmitted in any way without the publisher's prior written permission. This includes the use of mechanical or electronic techniques like photocopying and recording.

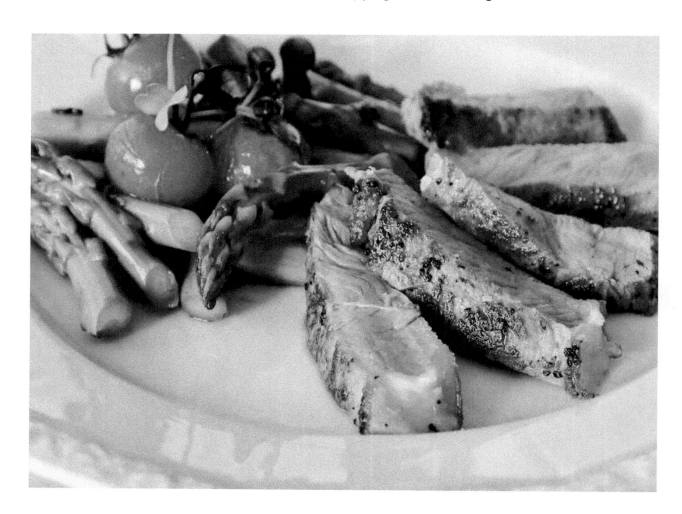

Table of Contents

James Cooper	0
Copyright Page	1
Table of Contents	2
Chapter 1:	**4**
Introduction to the Glucose Goddess Diet	**4**
1.1 Understanding Glucose and its Role in the Body	4
1.2 Benefits of the Glucose Goddess Diet	6
1.3 Getting Started: Essential Guidelines and Tips	8
Chapter 2:	**10**
Breakfast Recipes	**10**
2.1 Energizing Morning Smoothie Bowl	10
2.2 Gluten-Free Quinoa Pancakes	12
2.3 Veggie-Packed Omelet	14
2.4 Mushrooms and Swiss Omelette	16
2.5 Low Glycemic Banana Nut Pancake	18
Chapter 3:	**20**
Lunch and Dinner Recipes	**20**
3.1 Grilled Lemon-Herb Chicken with Roasted Vegetables	20
3.2 Quinoa-Stuffed Bell Peppers	22
3.3 Baked Salmon with Asparagus and Lemon-Dill Sauce	24
3.4 Chickpea and Spinach Curry	26
3.5 Greek Salad	28
Chapter 4:	**29**
Snacks and Appetizers	**29**
4.1 Fresh Veggie Sticks with Greek Yogurt Dip	29
4.2 Avocado and Black Bean Salsa	31
4.3 Roasted Sweet Potato Fries	33
Chapter 5:	**35**
Side Dishes	**35**
5.1 Quinoa and Roasted Vegetable Salad	35
5.2 Garlic and Parmesan Roasted Brussels Sprouts	37
5.3 Lemon-Herb Brown Rice Pilaf	39
Chapter 6:	**41**
Desserts and Sweet Treats	**41**
6.1 Raspberry Chia Seed Pudding	41
6.2 Flourless Chocolate Cake with Berry Compote	43
6.3 Coconut Macaroons	45

    Chapter 7: 47
    Beverages 47
        7.1 Fresh Green Juice Blend 47
        7.2 Homemade Iced Herbal Tea 49
        7.3 Detoxifying Infused Water 51

Chapter 8: 53

Meal Plans and Weekly Menus 53
        8.1 One-Week Glucose Goddess Meal Plan 53
        8.2 Grocery Shopping List for the Glucose Goddess Diet 55

Chapter 9: 57

Guidelines for the Glucose Goddess Diet's Success 57
        9.1 Mindful Eating and Portion Control 57
        9.2 Smart Carbohydrate Swaps 59
        9.3 Dining Out and Traveling on the Glucose Goddess Diet 61

Chapter 10: 63

Conclusion: 63
    Embracing a Healthier, Balanced Lifestyle 63

Chapter 1:

Introduction to the Glucose Goddess Diet

1.1 Understanding Glucose and its Role in the Body

The main source of energy for our bodies is a type of sugar called glucose. It is a simple carbohydrate that is found in many foods, including fruits, vegetables, grains, and dairy products. The glucose that is produced when we eat carbs is subsequently taken into the bloodstream by our bodies.

The level of glucose in our blood, known as blood glucose or blood sugar, needs to be carefully regulated to maintain optimal health. This regulation is primarily controlled by the hormone insulin, which is produced by the pancreas. Glucose can be used by cells to produce energy by being transported from the bloodstream into them with the aid of insulin.

The role of glucose in the body is essential for various bodily functions, including:

1. Energy Production: Glucose is the main fuel source for our cells and provides energy for all bodily processes, from basic cellular functions to physical activities.

2. Brain Function: The brain relies heavily on glucose for energy. It uses about 20% of the body's total glucose supply, making it crucial for cognitive functions and overall brain health.

3. Muscle Function: Muscles, including both skeletal and cardiac muscles, depend on glucose for contraction and movement.

4. Glycogen Storage: Excess glucose that is not immediately used for energy is converted into glycogen and stored in the liver and muscles. Glycogen serves as a readily available source of glucose when blood sugar levels drop.

5. Hormone Regulation: Blood glucose levels influence the release of several hormones, including insulin and glucagon, which work together to maintain glucose balance in the body.

However, consistently high blood glucose levels can lead to health issues, such as insulin resistance, type 2 diabetes, and increased risk of cardiovascular diseases. Therefore, it is important to consume carbohydrates in a balanced and controlled manner, choosing foods that provide sustained energy and have a minimal impact on blood sugar levels.

The Glucose Goddess Diet focuses on selecting nutrient-dense, low-glycemic foods that promote stable blood sugar levels, sustained energy, and overall well-being. By understanding the role of glucose in the body and making mindful dietary choices, you can support optimal health and vitality.

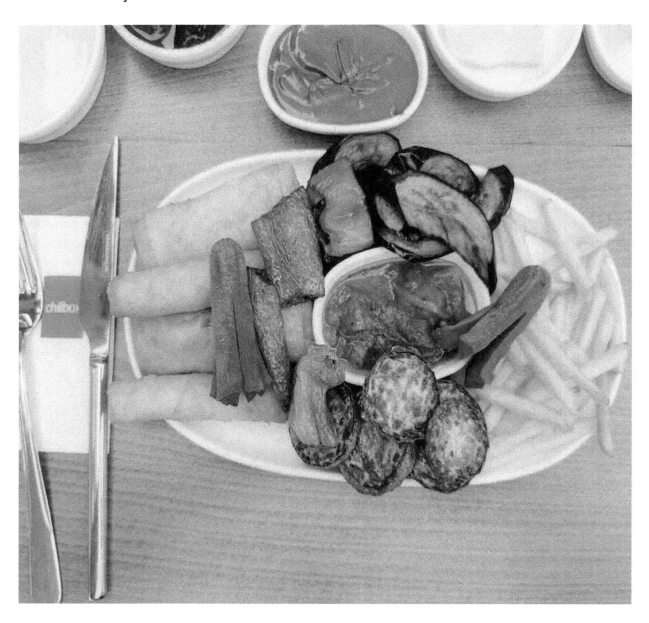

1.2 Benefits of the Glucose Goddess Diet

The Glucose Goddess Diet offers several potential benefits for individuals looking to improve their overall health and well-being. Here are some of the key benefits associated with following this diet:

1. Stable Blood Glucose Levels: The Glucose Goddess Diet focuses on consuming low-glycemic index (GI) foods, which release glucose slowly into the bloodstream. This helps maintain stable blood sugar levels, preventing spikes and crashes that can lead to fatigue, cravings, and mood swings.

2. Improved Energy Levels: By promoting stable blood glucose levels, the diet provides a consistent and sustained source of energy throughout the day. This can help prevent energy dips and provide a more balanced and steady supply of fuel for physical and mental activities.

3. Enhanced Weight Management: The diet emphasizes whole, nutrient-dense foods and portion control, which can support healthy weight management. The focus on low-GI foods and fiber-rich choices can increase satiety, reducing the likelihood of overeating and supporting weight loss or maintenance goals.

4. Balanced Hormonal Response: The Glucose Goddess Diet may help balance hormone levels, particularly insulin. By avoiding high-GI foods that can trigger insulin spikes, the diet can promote insulin sensitivity and improve overall hormonal balance in the body.

5. Reduced Risk of Chronic Diseases: Following a diet that maintains stable blood sugar levels and promotes a healthy weight can reduce the risk of chronic conditions such as type 2 diabetes, heart disease, and metabolic syndrome. By focusing on whole foods, the diet also provides essential nutrients and antioxidants that support overall health.

6. Enhanced Mental Clarity and Mood: Stable blood sugar levels can contribute to improved cognitive function, better focus, and enhanced mood stability. By avoiding blood sugar fluctuations, the Glucose Goddess Diet may help promote mental clarity and emotional well-being.

7. Improved Gut Health: The diet encourages the consumption of fiber-rich fruits, vegetables, and whole grains, which can support a healthy gut microbiome. A balanced gut microbiome is associated with improved digestion, nutrient absorption, and a strengthened immune system.

8. Variety and Flavorful Meals: The Glucose Goddess Diet promotes a balanced approach to eating, emphasizing whole, unprocessed foods and incorporating a wide variety of flavors,

textures, and colors. This encourages a more enjoyable and sustainable way of eating while still nourishing the body.

It's important to note that individual results may vary, and it's always recommended to consult with a healthcare professional or registered dietitian before starting any new dietary approach, especially if you have specific health conditions or dietary restrictions.

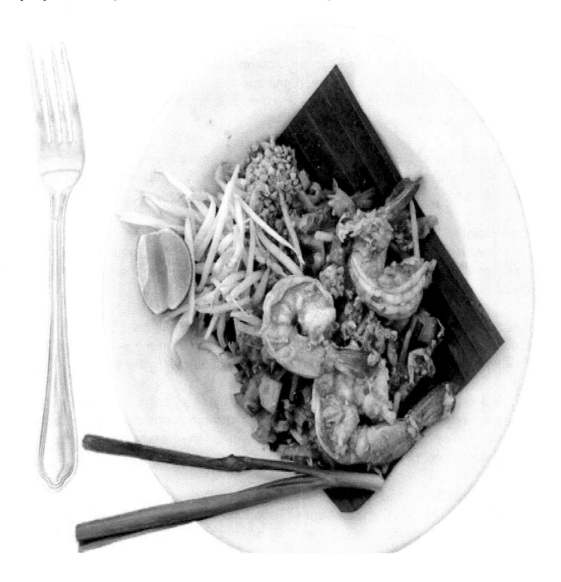

1.3 Getting Started: Essential Guidelines and Tips

When beginning the Glucose Goddess Diet, it's helpful to have some essential guidelines and tips to ensure a smooth transition and successful implementation. Consider the following important details:

1. Understand the Basics:
   - Familiarize yourself with the principles of the Glucose Goddess Diet, including the emphasis on low-glycemic index foods, balanced meals, and whole, unprocessed ingredients.
   - Educate yourself about the concept of glycemic index and glycemic load to make informed food choices that promote stable blood sugar levels.

2. Plan Your Meals:
   - Take time to plan your meals in advance to ensure you have balanced options readily available.
   - Create a meal plan for the week, including breakfast, lunch, dinner, and snacks, to avoid impulsive and unhealthy food choices.
   - Consider batch cooking and meal prepping to save time and have nutritious meals ready to enjoy throughout the week.

3. Focus on Whole Foods:
   - Choose entire, unprocessed foods instead, like fruits, vegetables, whole grains, lean meats, and healthy fats.
   - Minimize or avoid highly processed and sugary foods, including refined grains, sugary drinks, and snacks, as they can lead to rapid blood sugar spikes.

4. Balance Macronutrients:
   - Include a balance of macronutrients in each meal to promote satiety and stable blood sugar levels.
   - Make an effort to include a variety of complex carbohydrates, lean proteins, and healthy fats.
   - Examples of balanced meals include a quinoa salad with grilled chicken and mixed vegetables or a salmon fillet with roasted sweet potatoes and steamed greens.

5. Be Mindful of Portions:
   - To avoid overeating and control calorie intake, pay attention to portion sizes.
   - Use measuring cups or a food scale if needed to accurately portion your meals and snacks.

6. Stay Hydrated:
   - Consume enough water throughout the day to maintain your hydration and promote your general health.
   - Limit sugary beverages and opt for water, herbal tea, or infused water for hydration.

7. Practice Mindful Eating:

- Take your time and pay attention to your body's signals of hunger and fullness while you are eating.
   - Engage in mindful eating practices, such as savoring each bite, chewing slowly, and paying attention to the flavors and textures of your food.

8. Read Food Labels:
   - When purchasing packaged foods, read food labels carefully to identify added sugars and choose products with minimal processing and additives.

9. Seek Professional Guidance:
   - Consider consulting with a registered dietitian or healthcare professional who can provide personalized guidance, support, and monitor your progress on the Glucose Goddess Diet.

Remember, adopting a new dietary approach takes time and patience. It's essential to focus on progress rather than perfection, and to listen to your body's unique needs and responses along the way.

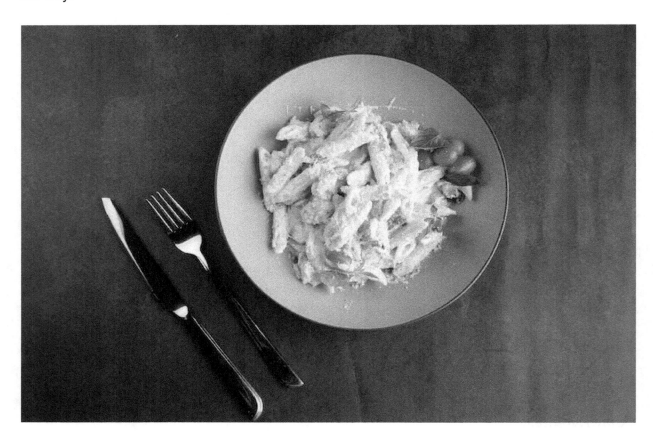

Chapter 2:

Breakfast Recipes

2.1 Energizing Morning Smoothie Bowl

Start your day off right with a delicious and nourishing Energizing Morning Smoothie Bowl. Packed with nutrients and natural sweetness, this bowl will provide you with the energy you need to kick-start your day. Here's the recipe:

Ingredients:

For the smoothie base:
- 1 frozen banana
- 1 cup of frozen berries, such as mixed berries, blueberries, or strawberries.
- 1/2 cup unsweetened almond milk (or any plant-based milk of your choice)
- 1 tablespoon chia seeds
- One tablespoon of peanut butter or almond butter
- 1/2 teaspoon honey or maple syrup (optional, for added sweetness)

Toppings:
- Sliced fresh fruits (such as berries, banana, kiwi, or mango)
- Granola or muesli
- Coconut flakes
- Nuts that have been chopped, such pecans, walnuts, or almonds
- Chia seed
- Honey or maple syrup drizzle, if desired

Instructions:

1. In a blender, combine the frozen banana, frozen berries, almond milk, chia seeds, almond butter or peanut butter, and sweetener (if desired). Blend until smooth and creamy. If needed, add a splash more almond milk to achieve the desired consistency.

2. Place a bowl with the smoothie mixture inside.

3. Arrange your desired toppings on top of the smoothie base. Get creative and use a variety of fresh fruits, granola, coconut flakes, chopped nuts, chia seeds, or a drizzle of honey or maple syrup.

4. Serve immediately and enjoy your energizing morning smoothie bowl!

Note: Feel free to customize your smoothie bowl with your favorite fruits, nuts, or seeds. You can also add additional superfood boosts like a scoop of protein powder, spirulina, or maca powder for an extra nutritional boost.

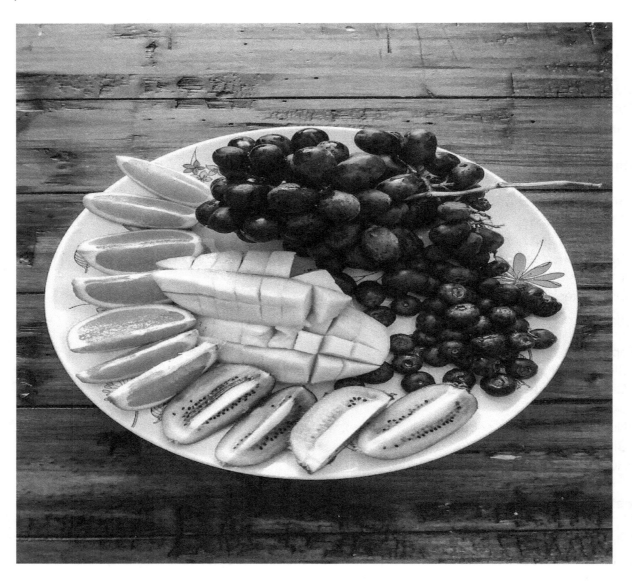

2.2 Gluten-Free Quinoa Pancakes

If you're looking for a delicious and gluten-free alternative to traditional pancakes, these Quinoa Pancakes are the perfect choice. Packed with protein and fiber, they are not only tasty but also provide a nutritious start to your day. Here's how to make them:

Ingredients:

- 1 cup cooked quinoa
- 1/2 cup gluten-free oat flour
- 2 tablespoons ground flaxseed
- 1 teaspoon baking powder
- 1/2 teaspoon ground cinnamon
- 1/4 teaspoon salt
- 1/2 cup unsweetened almond milk (or any plant-based milk of your choice)
- 2 tablespoons maple syrup (or your preferred sweetener)
- 1 teaspoon of vanilla extract
- Cooking spray or coconut oil for pan greasing

Optional toppings:
- Fresh berries
- Sliced bananas
- Maple syrup
- Nut butter

Instructions:

1. In a large bowl, combine the cooked quinoa, oat flour, ground flaxseed, baking powder, cinnamon, and salt. Stir until well mixed.

2. In a separate bowl, whisk together the almond milk, maple syrup, and vanilla extract.

3. Pour the wet ingredients into the dry ingredients and stir until well combined. The batter should be thick but pourable. If it's too thick, you can add a little more almond milk to achieve the desired consistency.

4. Set a nonstick skillet or griddle to medium heat. Grease the surface with coconut oil or cooking spray.

5. Spoon about 1/4 cup of the pancake batter onto the skillet for each pancake. Spread the batter into a circle using the back of a spoon.

6. Cook the pancakes for about 2-3 minutes on each side, or until golden brown. Flip carefully using a spatula.

7. Using the leftover batter, repeat the procedure, lubricating the pan as necessary.

8. Once all the pancakes are cooked, stack them on a plate and serve with your favorite toppings, such as fresh berries, sliced bananas, maple syrup, or nut butter.

9. Enjoy your gluten-free quinoa pancakes while they're warm and fluffy!

Note: You can prepare a larger batch of quinoa pancakes and store any leftovers in an airtight container in the refrigerator for a few days. Simply reheat them in a toaster or microwave before enjoying.

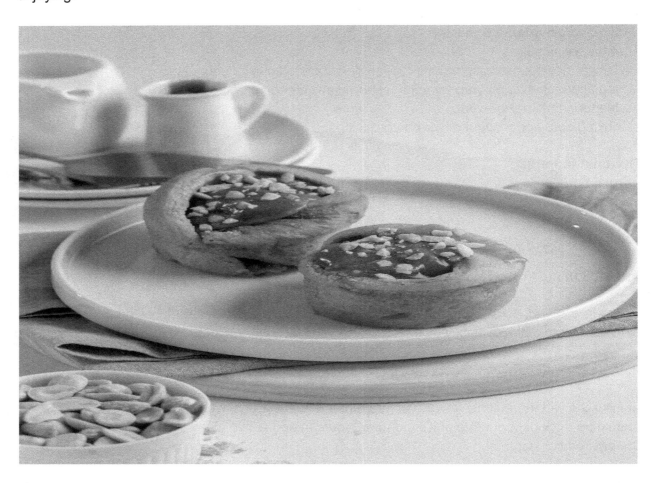

2.3 Veggie-Packed Omelet

A Veggie-Packed Omelet is a nutritious and flavorful way to start your day. This recipe combines eggs with a variety of colorful vegetables to create a delicious and satisfying meal. Feel free to customize the veggies based on your preferences and what's in season. Here's how to make it:

Ingredients:

- 3 large eggs
- 2 tablespoons milk (dairy or plant-based)
- Salt and pepper, to taste
- 1 tablespoon olive oil
- 1/4 cup diced onion
- 1/4 cup sliced bell peppers of any color
- 1/4 cup sliced mushrooms
- 1/4 cup chopped spinach or kale
- 2 tablespoons diced tomatoes
- 2 tablespoons shredded cheese (such as cheddar, feta, or goat cheese)
- Fresh herbs (optional, for garnish)

Instructions:

1. In a bowl, thoroughly blend the eggs, milk, salt, and pepper. Place aside.

2. In a nonstick skillet over medium heat, warm the olive oil.

3. Add the diced onion, bell peppers, and mushrooms to the skillet. The vegetables should be softened after 3 to 4 minutes of sautéing.

4. Add the chopped spinach or kale and diced tomatoes to the skillet. The greens should be cooked for a further 1-2 minutes or until wilted.

5. Pour the egg mixture over the cooked vegetables in the skillet. Give the eggs a brief moment to set.

6. Gently lift the edges of the omelet with a spatula, tilting the skillet to allow any uncooked eggs to flow to the edges.

7. Sprinkle the shredded cheese evenly over one half of the omelet.

8. Carefully fold the other half of the omelet over the cheese to create a half-moon shape. Press down gently with the spatula.

9. Cook for an additional 1-2 minutes, or until the cheese is melted and the omelet is cooked through.

10. Slide the omelet onto a plate, and if desired, garnish with fresh herbs like parsley or chives.

11. Serve your veggie-packed omelet hot and enjoy a nutritious breakfast!

Note: Feel free to add other vegetables like zucchini, broccoli, or asparagus to the omelet based on your preference. You can also experiment with different herbs, spices, or sauces to enhance the flavor.

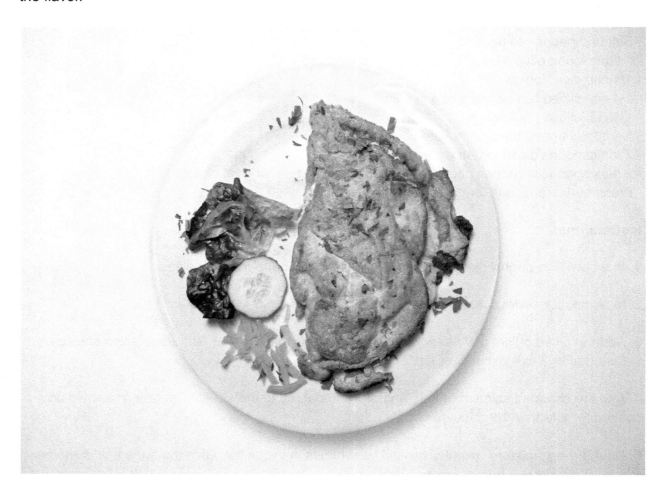

2.4 Mushrooms and Swiss Omelette

A Mushroom and Swiss Omelette is a delicious and satisfying breakfast option that combines the earthy flavors of mushrooms with the creamy goodness of Swiss cheese. Here's how to make it:

Ingredients:

- 3 large eggs
- 1/2 cup sliced mushrooms
- 1/4 cup shredded Swiss cheese
- 1 tablespoon butter
- Salt and pepper, to taste
- Fresh parsley, for garnish (optional)

Instructions:

1. In a bowl, vigorously beat the eggs.

2. Heat a non-stick skillet over medium heat. Add the butter and let it melt, ensuring the pan is evenly coated.

3. Add the sliced mushrooms to the skillet and sauté until they are tender and lightly browned, about 3-4 minutes. The mushrooms should be taken out of the skillet and put aside.

4. Pour the beaten eggs into the skillet, tilting the pan to spread the eggs evenly.

5. Gently raise the edges of the pan with a spatula as the eggs begin to set to let the uncooked eggs flow below.

6. Sprinkle the sautéed mushrooms evenly over one half of the omelette. Top with the shredded Swiss cheese.

7. Using the spatula, carefully fold the other half of the omelette over the filling.

8. Cook for another minute or two until the cheese is melted and the eggs are cooked through.

9. Slide the omelette onto a serving plate and garnish with fresh parsley if desired.

10. Serve the Mushroom and Swiss Omelette hot and enjoy a flavorful and protein-packed breakfast!

Note: Feel free to customize the omelette by adding other ingredients such as diced onions, bell peppers, or herbs like thyme or chives. Adjust the amount of mushrooms and cheese to your preference. This omelette pairs well with a side of whole grain toast or a fresh green salad.

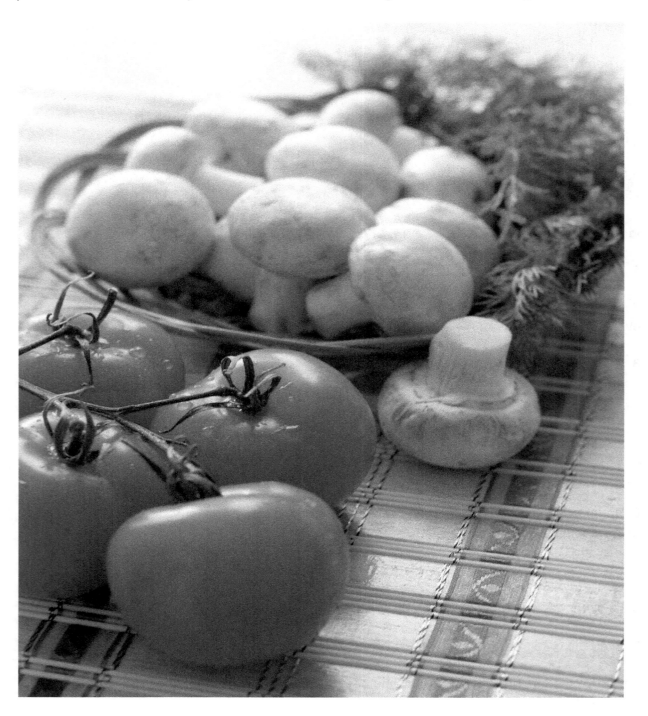

2.5 Low Glycemic Banana Nut Pancake

Ingredients:
- 1 ripe banana
- 2 eggs
- 1/4 cup almond flour
- 1/4 cup chopped walnuts or pecans
- 1/2 teaspoon baking powder
- 1/2 teaspoon vanilla extract
- Pinch of salt
- Coconut oil or butter for greasing the pan

Instructions:
1. In a mixing bowl, mash the ripe banana until it becomes smooth.
2. Add the eggs to the mashed banana and whisk together until well combined.
3. Stir in the almond flour, chopped nuts, baking powder, vanilla extract, and a pinch of salt. Mix all the ingredients together completely.
4. Preheat a griddle or nonstick skillet over medium heat. Add a small amount of coconut oil or butter to grease the surface.
5. Spoon about 1/4 cup of the pancake batter onto the heated skillet. Use the back of the spoon to spread it into a round shape.
6. Cook the pancake for about 2-3 minutes, or until bubbles start to form on the surface.
7. Flip the pancake and cook for an additional 1-2 minutes, or until it is cooked through and lightly browned.
8. Carry out step 7 with the remaining batter, adding more butter or coconut oil to the skillet as necessary.
9. Serve the low glycemic banana nut pancakes warm with toppings of your choice, such as fresh berries, a drizzle of honey or maple syrup (in moderation), or a dollop of Greek yogurt.

These pancakes are low glycemic because they use a ripe banana as a natural sweetener instead of processed sugar. The almond flour adds a nutty flavor and provides a lower carbohydrate alternative to traditional wheat flour. The chopped nuts add extra texture and healthy fats. Enjoy your delicious and healthier banana nut pancakes!

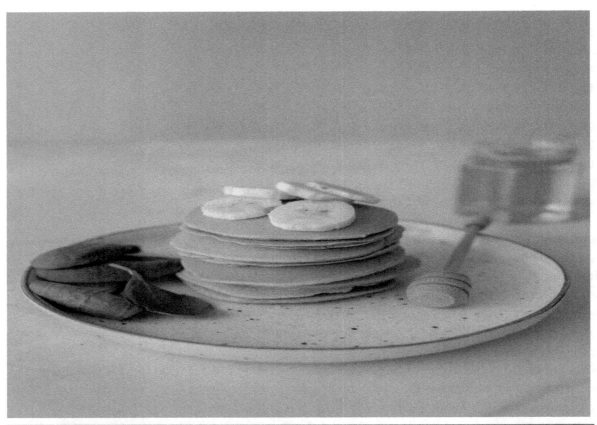
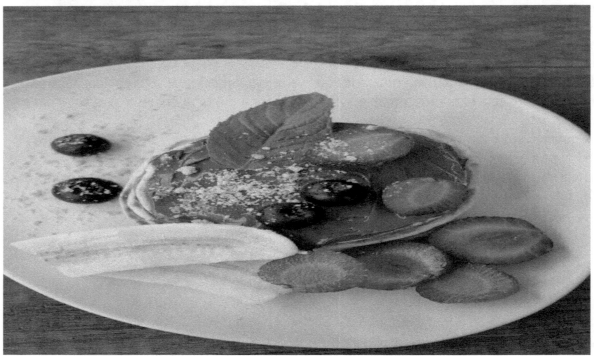

Chapter 3:

Lunch and Dinner Recipes

3.1 Grilled Lemon-Herb Chicken with Roasted Vegetables

This recipe combines juicy grilled chicken with flavorful roasted vegetables for a delicious and healthy meal. The lemon and herbs add a refreshing and aromatic touch. Here's how to make it:

Ingredients:

For the Lemon-Herb Chicken:
- 2 boneless, skinless chicken breasts
- Juice of 1 lemon
- Zest of 1 lemon
- 2 tablespoons olive oil
- 2 cloves garlic, minced
- 1 teaspoon dried thyme
- 1 teaspoon dried rosemary
- Salt and pepper, to taste

For the Roasted Vegetables:
- 2 cups mixed vegetables (such as bell peppers, zucchini, carrots, and red onions), cut into bite-sized pieces
- 2 tablespoons olive oil
- 1 teaspoon dried oregano
- 1 teaspoon dried basil
- Salt and pepper, to taste

Instructions:

1. Preheat the grill to medium-high heat.

2. Combine the olive oil, minced garlic, salt, pepper, dried thyme, dried rosemary, and lemon juice in a bowl. Make a good mixture.

3. Put the marinade in a shallow dish and cover the chicken breasts with it. Toss the coating on the chicken evenly. In the fridge, marinate it for at least 30 minutes and up to overnight.

4. While the chicken is marinating, preheat the oven to 425°F (220°C).

5. In a separate bowl, toss the mixed vegetables with olive oil, dried oregano, dried basil, salt, and pepper until well coated.

6. Spread the seasoned vegetables in a single layer on a baking sheet.

7. Roast the vegetables in the preheated oven for about 20-25 minutes or until they are tender and lightly browned, stirring once or twice during cooking.

8. While the vegetables are roasting, remove the chicken breasts from the marinade and discard the excess marinade.

9. Grill the chicken breasts on the preheated grill for about 6-8 minutes per side or until they reach an internal temperature of 165°F (74°C) and are cooked through. Depending on the thickness of the chicken breasts, cooking times may change.

10. Remove the grilled chicken from the grill and let it rest for a few minutes.

11. Slice the grilled lemon-herb chicken into thin strips.

12. Serve the grilled lemon-herb chicken alongside the roasted vegetables.

13. Enjoy your flavorful and nutritious grilled lemon-herb chicken with roasted vegetables!

Note: Feel free to adjust the seasoning and herbs according to your taste preferences. You can also add more vegetables or substitute them based on what you have available.

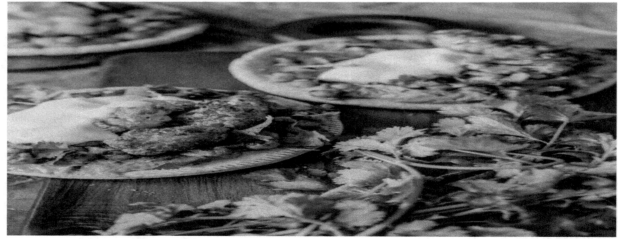

3.2 Quinoa-Stuffed Bell Peppers

Quinoa-Stuffed Bell Peppers are a nutritious and satisfying dish that combines the earthy flavors of quinoa with the sweetness of bell peppers. Packed with protein and veggies, this recipe makes a delicious and wholesome meal. Here's how to make it:

Ingredients:

- 4 bell peppers (any color)
- 1 cup cooked quinoa
- 1 tablespoon olive oil
- 1 small onion, diced
- 2 cloves garlic, minced
- 1 carrot, diced
- 1 zucchini, diced
- 1 cup diced tomatoes (fresh or canned)
- 1 teaspoon dried oregano
- 1 teaspoon dried basil
- 1/2 teaspoon ground cumin
- Salt and pepper, to taste
- Optional: 1/2 cup of shredded cheese, preferably mozzarella or cheddar
- Fresh cilantro or parsley, chopped (for garnish)

Instructions:

1. Preheat the oven to 375°F (190°C).

2. Slice off the tops of the bell peppers and remove the seeds and membranes from the inside. Set the bell peppers aside.

3. Place a large skillet over medium heat and warm the olive oil. Add the minced garlic and onion, both diced. Sauté the onion until it turns transparent and smells good.

4. Include in the skillet the diced carrot and zucchini. Vegetables should be cooked for a few minutes until they start to soften.

5. Stir in the cooked quinoa, diced tomatoes, dried oregano, dried basil, ground cumin, salt, and pepper. To thoroughly incorporate all ingredients, stir well.

6. Cook the mixture for a few more minutes until the flavors meld together and the vegetables are tender.

7. Fill each bell pepper with the quinoa and vegetable mixture, packing it tightly. You can sprinkle some shredded cheese on top if desired.

8. Place the stuffed bell peppers in a baking dish, standing upright.

9. Bake in the preheated oven for about 25-30 minutes, or until the bell peppers are tender and slightly charred on the outside.

10. Remove the stuffed bell peppers from the oven and let them cool for a few minutes.

11. Garnish with freshly chopped parsley or cilantro.

12. Serve the quinoa-stuffed bell peppers as a main course or a side dish.

13. Enjoy your flavorful and wholesome quinoa-stuffed bell peppers!

Note: You can customize this recipe by adding other vegetables, spices, or herbs to the quinoa stuffing based on your preferences. For added protein, you can also mix in cooked chicken, tofu, or beans.

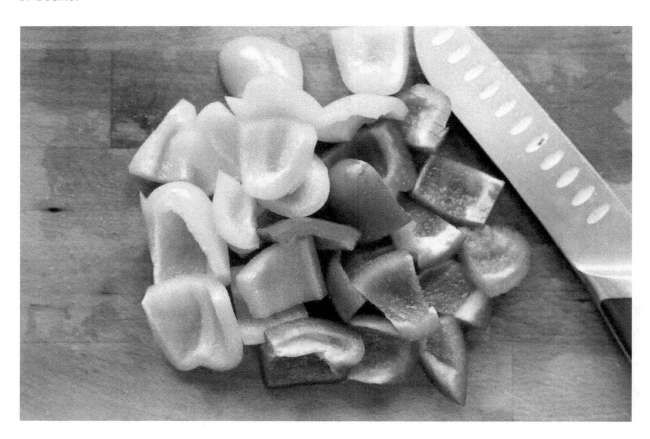

3.3 Baked Salmon with Asparagus and Lemon-Dill Sauce

This recipe features tender and flavorful baked salmon accompanied by roasted asparagus and a tangy lemon-dill sauce. It's a nutritious and delicious dish that showcases the natural flavors of the ingredients. Here's how to make it:

Ingredients:

For the Baked Salmon:
- 4 salmon fillets
- 2 tablespoons olive oil
- Salt and pepper, to taste
- Lemon slices, for garnish

For the Roasted Asparagus:
- 1 bunch asparagus, woody ends trimmed
- 1 tablespoon olive oil
- Salt and pepper, to taste

For the Lemon-Dill Sauce:
- 1/2 cup plain Greek yogurt
- Zest and juice of 1 lemon
- 1 teaspoon dried dill or 1 tablespoon of fresh dill diced.
- Salt and pepper, to taste

Instructions:

1. Preheat the oven to 400°F (200°C).

2. Place the salmon fillets on a baking sheet lined with parchment paper or foil. Drizzle olive oil over the salmon and season with salt and pepper to taste. The fillets should be covered with lemon slices.

3. Toss the trimmed asparagus with olive oil, salt, and pepper on a separate baking sheet.

4. Place both the salmon and asparagus in the preheated oven. Bake for about 12-15 minutes, or until the salmon is cooked through and flakes easily with a fork, and the asparagus is tender and slightly charred.

5. While the salmon and asparagus are baking, prepare the lemon-dill sauce. In a small bowl, whisk together the Greek yogurt, lemon zest, lemon juice, chopped dill, salt, and pepper. Adapt the seasoning to your personal tastes.

6. Once the salmon and asparagus are done, remove them from the oven.

7. Serve the baked salmon on a plate alongside the roasted asparagus. Drizzle the lemon-dill sauce over the salmon and asparagus.

8. Garnish with additional lemon slices and fresh dill, if desired.

9. Enjoy your delicious baked salmon with asparagus and tangy lemon-dill sauce!

Note: Feel free to adjust the seasoning and herbs based on your preferences. You can also serve this dish with a side of cooked quinoa, rice, or a fresh salad for a complete and balanced meal.

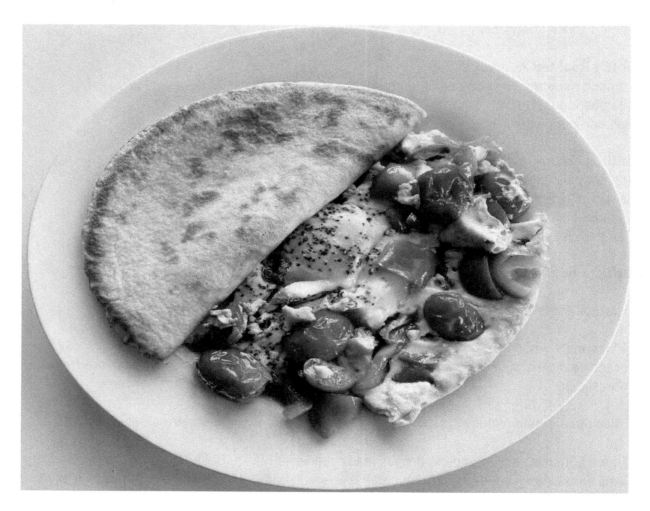

3.4 Chickpea and Spinach Curry

Chickpea and Spinach Curry is a flavorful and nourishing vegetarian dish that combines protein-rich chickpeas with vibrant spinach and aromatic spices. It's a satisfying meal that can be enjoyed with rice or naan bread. Here's how to make it:

Ingredients:

- 1 tablespoon oil (such as olive oil or coconut oil)
- 1 onion, finely chopped
- 3 cloves garlic, minced
- 1 teaspoon grated ginger
- 1 tablespoon curry powder
- 1 teaspoon ground cumin
- 1 teaspoon ground coriander
- 1/2 teaspoon turmeric
- A quarter-teaspoon of cayenne pepper (optional; for extra heat).
- 1 can (15 oz) washed and drained chickpeas
- 1 can (14 oz) diced tomatoes
- 1 cup vegetable broth or water
- 2 cups fresh spinach leaves
- 1/2 cup coconut milk
- Salt and pepper, to taste
- Fresh cilantro, chopped (for garnish)

Instructions:

1. In a big skillet or pot, heat the oil over medium heat.

2. Place the chopped onion in the skillet and cook it for a few minutes, or until it softens and transparent.

3. Include the grated ginger and minced garlic in the skillet. Cook until aromatic for one more minute.

4. Fill the skillet with the curry powder, ground cumin, ground coriander, ground turmeric, and cayenne pepper (if using). For approximately a minute, stir and sauté the spices to toast them and bring out their aromas.

5. Fill the skillet with the washed and drained chickpeas. Stir to distribute the spices throughout.

6. Pour in the diced tomatoes (with their juices) and vegetable broth or water. Bring the mixture to a simmer and let it cook for about 10 minutes, allowing the flavors to meld together and the chickpeas to absorb the flavors.

7. Stir in the fresh spinach leaves and coconut milk. The spinach should wilt after a further 2 to 3 minutes of cooking.

8. Season the curry with salt and pepper to taste. Adjust the seasoning and spice level according to your preference.

9. Remove the skillet from the heat.

10. Serve the chickpea and spinach curry over cooked rice or with warm naan bread.

11. Garnish with freshly chopped cilantro.

12. Enjoy your delicious and comforting chickpea and spinach curry!

Note: You can customize this recipe by adding other vegetables such as diced bell peppers, carrots, or potatoes. You can also adjust the consistency of the curry by adding more coconut milk or vegetable broth if desired.

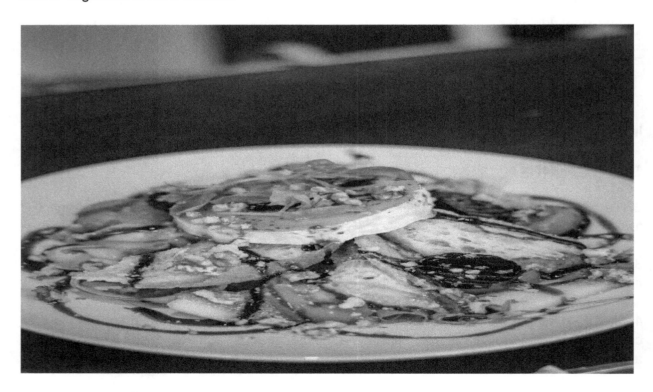

3.5 Greek Salad

Certainly! Below are simple and easy to use recipe for a classic Greek salad:

Ingredients:
- 2 large tomatoes, cut into wedges
- 1 cucumber, sliced
- 1 small red onion, thinly sliced
- 1 green bell pepper, seeded and sliced
- 1/2 cup Kalamata olives
- 1/2 cup crumbled feta cheese
- 2 tablespoons extra-virgin olive oil
- 1 tablespoon red wine vinegar
- 1 teaspoon dried oregano
- Salt and pepper to taste

Instructions:
1. In a large salad bowl, combine the tomato wedges, cucumber slices, red onion slices, bell pepper slices, and Kalamata olives.
2. In a small bowl, whisk together the extra-virgin olive oil, red wine vinegar, dried oregano, salt, and pepper.
3. Drizzle the dressing over the salad and gently toss to coat all the ingredients evenly.
4. Sprinkle the crumbled feta cheese on top of the salad.
5. Allow the flavors to mingle together by letting the Greek salad sit for a while.
6. Serve the salad as a refreshing side dish or add grilled chicken or shrimp to make it a complete meal.
7. Enjoy your Greek salad!

You are welcome to change the ingredients and amounts to suit your tastes. You can also add additional ingredients such as fresh herbs like parsley or mint, or even some chopped avocado for extra creaminess. Enjoy this light and flavorful Mediterranean salad!

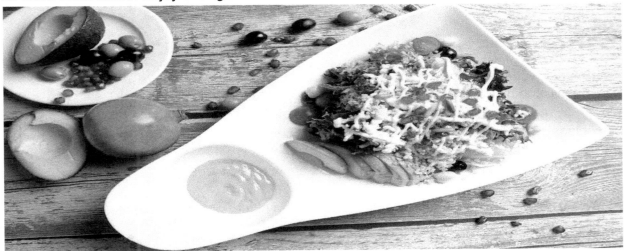

Chapter 4:

Snacks and Appetizers

4.1 Fresh Veggie Sticks with Greek Yogurt Dip

Fresh Veggie Sticks with Greek Yogurt Dip is a healthy and refreshing snack option that combines crunchy vegetables with a creamy and flavorful dip. It's a great way to increase your vegetable intake and enjoy a nutritious snack. Here's how to make it:

Ingredients:

For the Greek Yogurt Dip:
- 1 cup Greek yogurt
- 1 tablespoon lemon juice
- 1 clove garlic, minced
- 1 teaspoon dried dill or 1 tablespoon of fresh dill diced.
- Salt and pepper, to taste

For the Veggie Sticks:
- Carrot sticks
- Celery sticks
- Cucumber sticks
- Bell pepper strips
- Cherry tomatoes

Instructions:

1. In a bowl, combine the Greek yogurt, lemon juice, minced garlic, chopped dill, salt, and pepper. All materials should be completely blended after mixing. To suit your tastes, adjust the seasoning.

2. Wash and prepare the vegetables by cutting them into sticks or strips.

3. Arrange the vegetable sticks and strips on a serving platter or individual plates.

4. Serve the Greek yogurt dip alongside the veggie sticks.

5. Dip the vegetable sticks into the Greek yogurt dip and enjoy!

Note: Feel free to add other vegetables such as radishes, broccoli florets, or snap peas to the assortment based on your preferences. You can also customize the dip by adding herbs like parsley, chives, or basil for extra flavor. Enjoy this nutritious snack as a light appetizer or as a side dish with your meals.

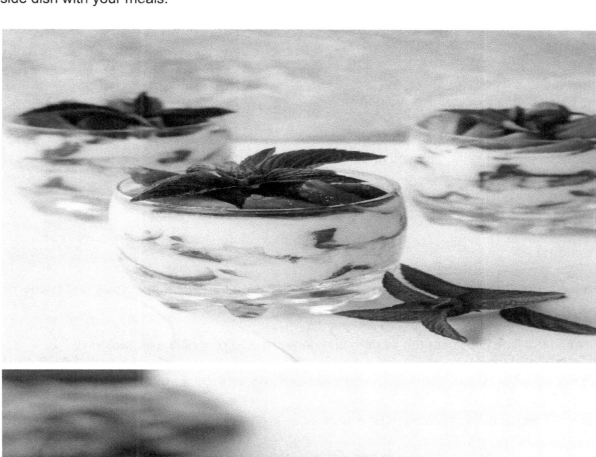

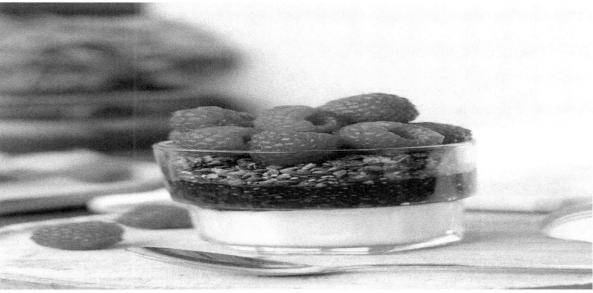

4.2 Avocado and Black Bean Salsa

Avocado and Black Bean Salsa is a vibrant and flavorful combination of creamy avocado, hearty black beans, juicy tomatoes, and zesty lime juice. It's a versatile salsa that can be enjoyed as a dip, topping for grilled meats or tacos, or even as a salad. Here's how to make it:

Ingredients:

- 1 ripe avocado, diced
- 1 cup black beans, cooked and drained
- 1 cup diced tomatoes
- 1/4 cup diced red onion
- 1 jalapeño pepper, seeds removed and finely diced (optional, for heat)
- Juice of 1 lime
- 2 tablespoons chopped fresh cilantro
- Salt and pepper, to taste

Instructions:

1. In a bowl, combine the diced avocado, black beans, diced tomatoes, red onion, and jalapeño pepper (if using).

2. Squeeze the lime juice over the mixture and gently toss to coat all the ingredients.

3. Add the chopped cilantro and season with salt and pepper to taste. Mix well.

4. Taste and adjust the seasoning or lime juice as desired.

5. Cover the bowl with plastic wrap or transfer the salsa to an airtight container. To give the flavors a chance to mingle, chill for at least 30 minutes.
6. Just before serving, give the salsa a gentle stir.

7. Serve the avocado and black bean salsa as a dip with tortilla chips or as a topping for grilled meats, tacos, or salads.

8. Enjoy the fresh and zesty flavors of the avocado and black bean salsa!

Note: You can customize this salsa by adding other ingredients like corn, diced bell peppers, or chopped jalapeños for extra heat. You can also adjust the amount of lime juice and cilantro based on your taste preferences. This salsa is best enjoyed fresh, but if you have leftovers, store them in an airtight container in the refrigerator for up to two days.

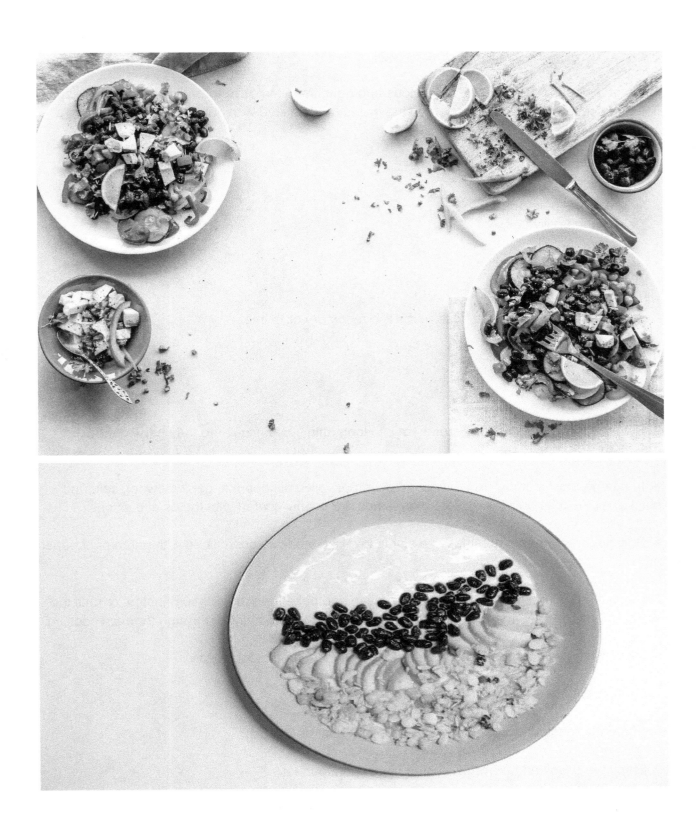

4.3 Roasted Sweet Potato Fries

Roasted sweet potato fries are a delicious and healthier alternative to traditional french fries. They are crispy on the outside, soft on the inside, and packed with natural sweetness. Here's how to make them:

Ingredients:

- 2 large sweet potatoes
- 2 tablespoons olive oil
- 1 teaspoon paprika
- 1/2 teaspoon garlic powder
- 1/2 teaspoon salt
- 1/4 teaspoon black pepper
- As an optional garnish, use fresh herbs like rosemary or thyme.

Instructions:

1. Preheat the oven to 425°F (220°C).

2. Peel the sweet potatoes and cut them into long, thin strips, similar to the shape of french fries.

3. In a large bowl, combine the sweet potato strips, olive oil, paprika, garlic powder, salt, and black pepper. Toss until the sweet potato strips are evenly coated with the oil and spices.

4. Spread the sweet potato strips in a single layer on a baking sheet lined with parchment paper or foil.

5. Place the baking sheet in the preheated oven and bake for about 25-30 minutes, or until the sweet potato fries are crispy and golden brown, flipping them halfway through for even cooking.

6. Remove the sweet potato fries from the oven and let them cool slightly.

7. Garnish with fresh herbs, if desired.

8. Serve the roasted sweet potato fries as a side dish or a snack.

9. Enjoy the crispy and flavorful roasted sweet potato fries!

Note: You can experiment with different seasonings and spices according to your taste preferences. Feel free to add a sprinkle of cayenne pepper for some heat or a dash of cinnamon for a touch of sweetness. Serve the fries with your favorite dipping sauce, such as ketchup, aioli, or a spicy mayo.

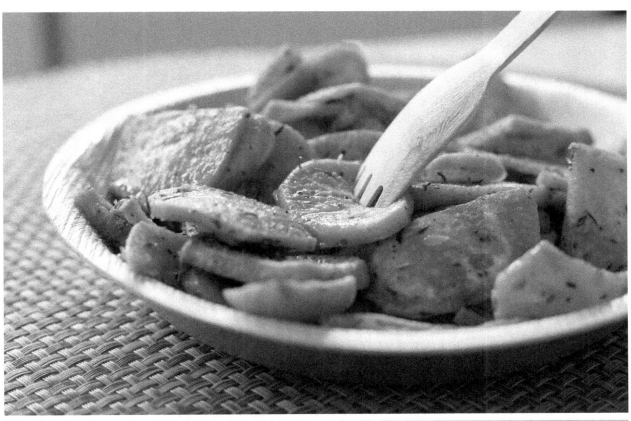
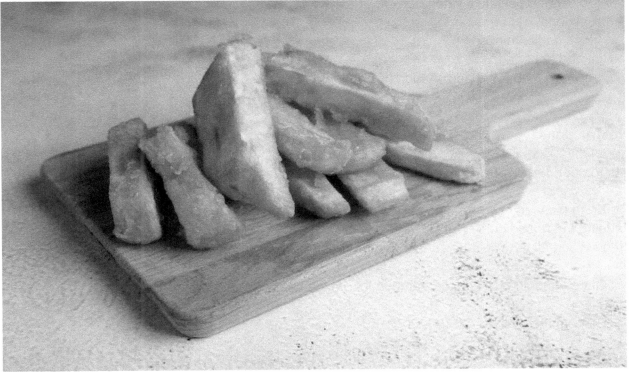

Chapter 5:

Side Dishes

5.1 Quinoa and Roasted Vegetable Salad

Quinoa and Roasted Vegetable Salad is a hearty and nutritious dish that combines fluffy quinoa with a variety of roasted vegetables, creating a flavorful and satisfying salad. It works well as a side dish or light supper. This is how to do it:

Ingredients:

- 1 cup quinoa
- 2 cups water or vegetable broth
- 2 cups mixed roasted vegetables (such as bell peppers, zucchini, eggplant, cherry tomatoes, and red onions), cut into bite-sized pieces
- 2 tablespoons olive oil
- 1 tablespoon balsamic vinegar
- 1 teaspoon Dijon mustard
- 1 clove garlic, minced
- Salt and pepper, to taste
- Finely chopped fresh herbs, such as parsley or basil,

Instructions:

1. To get rid of any bitterness, thoroughly rinse the quinoa in cold water.

2. Bring the water or vegetable broth to a boil in a saucepan. Turn down the heat to low before adding the rinsed quinoa. Cover and simmer for about 15-20 minutes, or until the quinoa is tender and all the liquid has been absorbed.

3. Once the quinoa is cooked, remove it from the heat and let it cool slightly.

4. Preheat the oven to 425°F (220°C).

5. Toss the mixed roasted vegetables with olive oil, salt, and pepper on a baking sheet.

6. Roast the vegetables in the preheated oven for about 20-25 minutes, or until they are tender and lightly browned, stirring once or twice during cooking.

7. In a small bowl, whisk together the balsamic vinegar, Dijon mustard, minced garlic, salt, and pepper.

8. In a large serving bowl, combine the cooked quinoa, roasted vegetables, and the dressing. Toss everything with care so that it is everything uniformly coated.

9. Taste the food and, if necessary, correct the seasoning.

10. Garnish with freshly chopped herbs, such as parsley or basil.

11. Serve the quinoa and roasted vegetable salad warm or chilled.

12. Enjoy the flavorful and nutritious quinoa and roasted vegetable salad!

Note: You can customize this salad by adding other ingredients such as feta cheese, toasted nuts or seeds, dried cranberries, or a squeeze of lemon juice for a tangy twist. This salad can be enjoyed on its own or as a side dish with grilled chicken, fish, or tofu. The refrigerator is a good place to keep leftovers for a few days if they are sealed tightly.

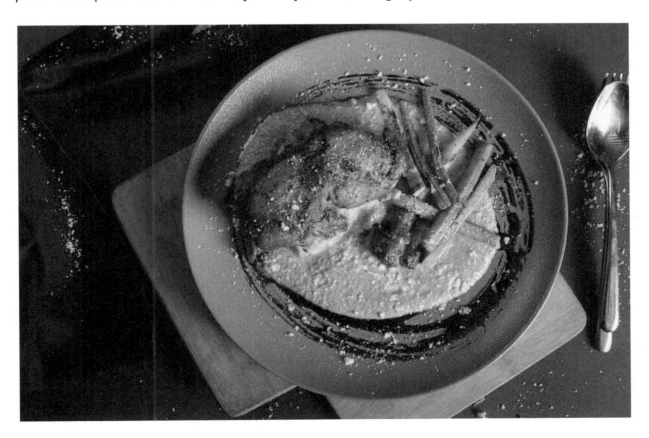

5.2 Garlic and Parmesan Roasted Brussels Sprouts

Garlic and Parmesan Roasted Brussels Sprouts are a flavorful and delicious side dish that brings out the natural sweetness and nuttiness of Brussels sprouts. The combination of roasted garlic and savory Parmesan cheese adds a delightful twist. Here's how to make them:

Ingredients:

- 1 pound Brussels sprouts, trimmed and halved
- 3 tablespoons olive oil
- 4 cloves garlic, minced
- 1/4 cup grated Parmesan cheese
- Salt and pepper, to taste

Instructions:

1. Preheat the oven to 400°F (200°C).

2. In a large bowl, toss the halved Brussels sprouts with olive oil, minced garlic, salt, and pepper until well coated.

3. Spread the Brussels sprouts in a single layer on a baking sheet lined with parchment paper or foil.

4. Roast the Brussels sprouts in the preheated oven for about 20-25 minutes, or until they are tender and lightly browned, stirring once or twice during cooking.

5. Remove the Brussels sprouts from the oven and sprinkle the grated Parmesan cheese over them. Toss gently to coat the Brussels sprouts evenly with the cheese.

6. Return the baking sheet to the oven and roast for an additional 5 minutes, or until the cheese is melted and slightly golden.

7. Remove from the oven and let the roasted Brussels sprouts cool slightly.

8. Serve the garlic and Parmesan roasted Brussels sprouts as a side dish or appetizer.

9. Enjoy the flavorful and savory garlic and Parmesan roasted Brussels sprouts!

Note: You can modify the proportions of garlic and Parmesan cheese to suit your tastes. For added variation, you can also sprinkle some lemon zest or red pepper flakes over the roasted Brussels sprouts for a tangy or spicy kick. This dish pairs well with a variety of main courses, such as roasted chicken, grilled steak, or baked salmon.

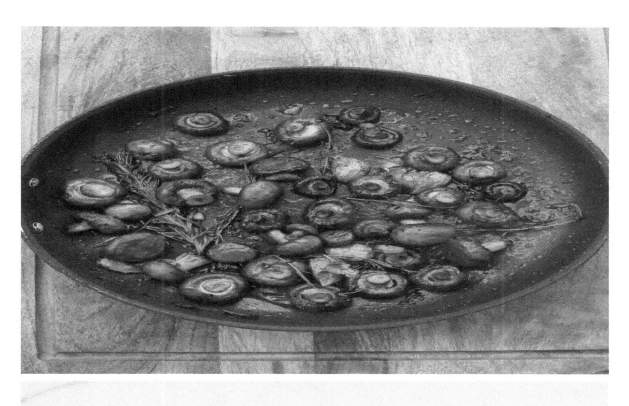
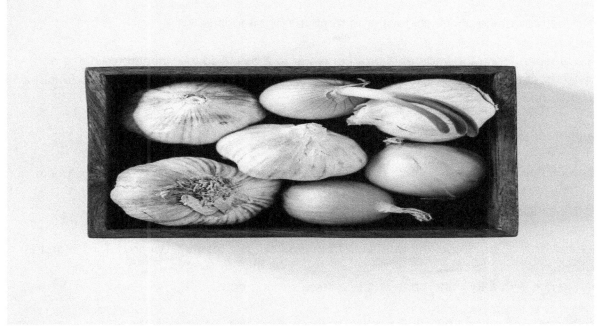

5.3 Lemon-Herb Brown Rice Pilaf

Lemon-Herb Brown Rice Pilaf is a fragrant and flavorful side dish that combines the nuttiness of brown rice with the freshness of lemon and aromatic herbs. It's a healthy and delicious accompaniment to a variety of main courses. Here's how to make it:

Ingredients:

- 1 cup brown rice
- 2 cups vegetable broth or water
- Zest and juice of 1 lemon
- 2 teaspoons of freshly chopped herbs, such as parsley, dill, or basil
- 1 tablespoon olive oil
- 1 small onion, finely chopped
- 2 cloves garlic, minced
- Salt and pepper, to taste

Instructions:

1. Rinse the brown rice under cold water to remove any impurities.

2. In a saucepan, bring the vegetable broth or water to a boil. Add the rinsed brown rice and reduce the heat to low. Cover and simmer for about 40-45 minutes, or until the rice is tender and all the liquid has been absorbed.

3. In a another skillet over medium heat, warm the olive oil while the rice is cooking.

4. Add the finely chopped onion to the skillet and sauté until it becomes soft and translucent.

5. Add the minced garlic to the skillet and cook for another minute until fragrant.

6. Once the brown rice is cooked, remove it from the heat and let it sit, covered, for 5 minutes.

7. Fluff the rice with a fork and transfer it to a large serving bowl.

8. Add the sautéed onion and garlic mixture to the bowl of rice, along with the lemon zest, lemon juice, chopped herbs, salt, and pepper.

9. Gently toss all the ingredients together until well combined.

10. Taste and adjust the seasoning or lemon juice if needed.

11. Serve the lemon-herb brown rice pilaf as a side dish with your favorite main course.

12. Enjoy the fragrant and flavorful lemon-herb brown rice pilaf!

Note: Feel free to customize this recipe by adding other ingredients like toasted nuts, dried fruits, or sautéed vegetables to the pilaf for added texture and flavor. You can also experiment with different combinations of herbs based on your preference. The refrigerator is a good place to keep leftovers for a few days if they are sealed tightly.

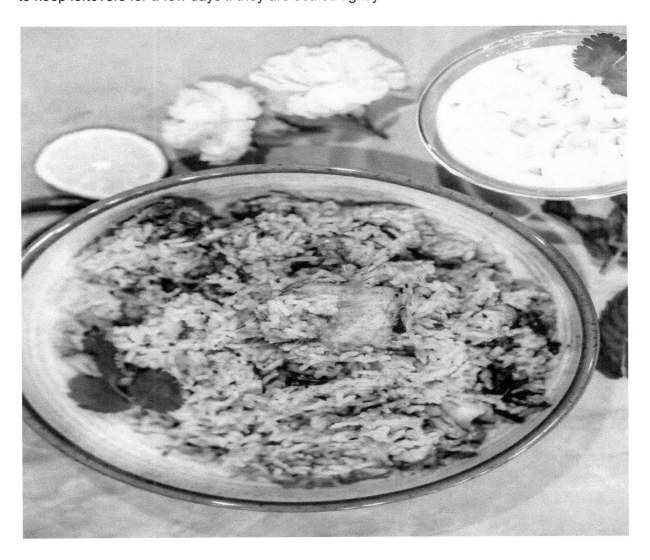

Chapter 6:

Desserts and Sweet Treats

6.1 Raspberry Chia Seed Pudding

Raspberry Chia Seed Pudding is a delicious and nutritious dessert or breakfast option that is packed with fiber, antioxidants, and omega-3 fatty acids. The combination of creamy chia seeds and tangy raspberries creates a delightful treat. Here's how to make it:

Ingredients:

- 1 cup raspberries (fresh or frozen)
- One cup of unsweetened almond milk (or other plant-based milk of your preference)
- 3 tablespoons chia seeds
- 1-2 tablespoons maple syrup or honey (optional, for added sweetness)
- 1/2 teaspoon vanilla extract
- Optional toppings: Fresh raspberries, sliced almonds, shredded coconut, or granola

Instructions:

1. Puree the raspberries in a blender or food processor until they are smooth.

2. In a bowl or jar, combine the raspberry puree, almond milk, chia seeds, maple syrup or honey (if using), and vanilla extract. To make sure the chia seeds are dispersed equally, stir thoroughly.

3. Let the mixture sit for about 5 minutes to allow the chia seeds to start absorbing the liquid. Give it a good stir again to prevent clumping.

4. Cover the bowl or jar and refrigerate for at least 2 hours, or overnight, to allow the chia seeds to fully gel and thicken.

5. After the pudding has set, give it a stir to break up any clumps and ensure a smooth consistency.

6. Divide the raspberry chia seed pudding into serving bowls or jars.

7. If desired, top each serving with fresh raspberries, sliced almonds, shredded coconut, or granola for added texture and flavor.

8. Serve the raspberry chia seed pudding chilled.

9. Enjoy the creamy and nutritious raspberry chia seed pudding as a dessert or a healthy breakfast!

Note: You can customize this recipe by using different types of berries or adding other flavorings such as cinnamon or cocoa powder. Adjust the sweetness level to your taste preferences by adding more or less maple syrup or honey. This pudding can be stored in the refrigerator for up to 3-4 days.

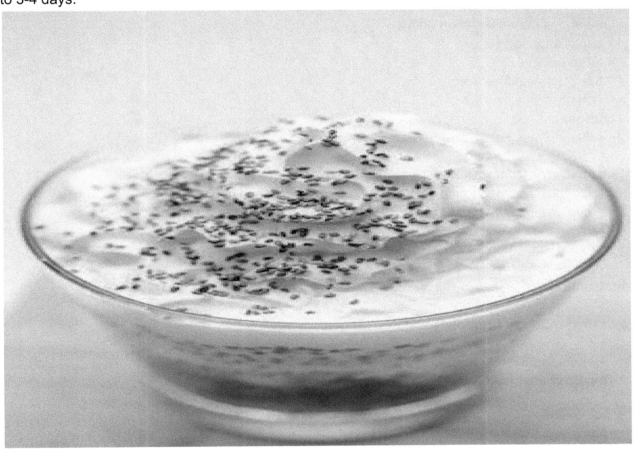

6.2 Flourless Chocolate Cake with Berry Compote

Flourless Chocolate Cake with Berry Compote is a decadent and rich dessert that combines the lusciousness of chocolate cake with the vibrant flavors of a sweet and tangy berry compote. It's a gluten-free treat that will satisfy any chocolate lover's cravings. Here's how to make it:

Ingredients:

For the Flourless Chocolate Cake:
- 8 ounces dark chocolate, chopped
- One cup of cubed unsalted butter
- 1 cup granulated sugar
- 4 large eggs
- 1 teaspoon vanilla extract
- Pinch of salt
- **Optional:**
 For dusting, use cocoa powder or powdered sugar.

For the Berry Compote:
- 2 cups mixed berries (such as strawberries, raspberries, blueberries)
- 1/4 cup granulated sugar
- 2 tablespoons water
- 1 tablespoon lemon juice

Instructions:

For the Flourless Chocolate Cake:

1. Preheat the oven to 325°F (160°C). A 9-inch round cake pan should be greased and lined with parchment paper on the bottom.

2. Melt the butter and chopped chocolate in a heatproof dish set over a pan of simmering water. Stir occasionally until the mixture is smooth and well-combined. Take it off the fire and give it a minute to cool.

3. In a separate large mixing bowl, whisk together the granulated sugar, eggs, vanilla extract, and salt until well combined.

4. Gradually pour the melted chocolate mixture into the sugar and egg mixture, whisking constantly until smooth and incorporated.

5. Pour the batter into the prepared cake pan and smooth the top with a spatula.

6. Bake in the preheated oven for about 30-35 minutes or until a toothpick inserted into the center comes out with a few moist crumbs.

7. Remove the cake from the oven and let it cool in the pan for 10 minutes. After that, move it to a wire rack to finish cooling.

8. Once the cake is cooled, you can dust it with cocoa powder or powdered sugar for an optional decorative touch.

For the Berry Compote:

1. In a saucepan, combine the mixed berries, granulated sugar, water, and lemon juice. Stir well.

2. Over medium heat, bring the mixture to a simmer. Cook for about 10-15 minutes, stirring occasionally, until the berries have softened and released their juices.

3. Remove the compote from the heat and let it cool slightly. As it cools, the compote will get thicker.

To Serve:

1. Slice the flourless chocolate cake into desired portions and place each slice on a serving plate.

2. Spoon a generous amount of the berry compote over each slice of cake.

3. Optionally, garnish with additional fresh berries or a dusting of powdered sugar.

4. Serve the flourless chocolate cake with berry compote and enjoy the indulgent and delightful combination!

Note: The cake can be stored in an airtight container at room temperature for a few days. The berry compote can be stored in the refrigerator for up to a week. Warm the compote slightly before serving if it thickens too much in the refrigerator.

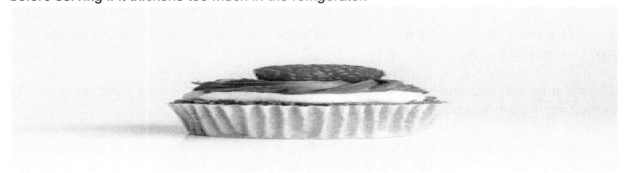

6.3 Coconut Macaroons

Coconut macaroons are sweet and chewy treats that are simple to make and bursting with coconut flavor. These delightful cookies are perfect for coconut lovers and make a great addition to any dessert platter. Here's how to make them:

Ingredients:

- 3 cups shredded coconut (sweetened or unsweetened)
- 3/4 cup sweetened condensed milk
- 2 teaspoons vanilla extract
- 2 large egg whites
- 1/4 teaspoon salt
- Optional: Chocolate for drizzling or dipping (melted)

Instructions:

1. Set the oven temperature to 325°F (160°C). Use silicone mat or parchment paper to line a baking sheet.

2. In a large mixing bowl, combine the shredded coconut, sweetened condensed milk, and vanilla extract. All materials should be completely blended after mixing.

3. In a separate bowl, beat the egg whites with salt until they reach stiff peaks. Both a hand mixer and a stand mixer with the whisk attachment are acceptable.

4. Gently incorporate the egg whites that have been beaten into the coconut mixture.Be careful not to overmix; the mixture should be sticky and well combined.

5. Using a spoon or a cookie scoop, portion the coconut mixture onto the prepared baking sheet, forming small mounds of about 1.5 inches in diameter. Give them some room to spread by separating them.

6. Bake in the preheated oven for about 15-20 minutes, or until the coconut macaroons are golden brown on the edges.

7. Remove from the oven and let the macaroons cool on the baking sheet for a few minutes. After that, move them to a wire rack to finish cooling.

8. If desired, melt some chocolate and drizzle or dip the cooled macaroons for an extra touch of sweetness and flavor. Allow the chocolate to set before serving.

9. Serve the coconut macaroons as a delightful treat for dessert or a snack.

10. Enjoy the sweet and chewy coconut macaroons!

The coconut macaroons can be kept at room temperature for a few days in an airtight container. Place them in the refrigerator for longer storage. Also freezer-safe for a month, these cookies.

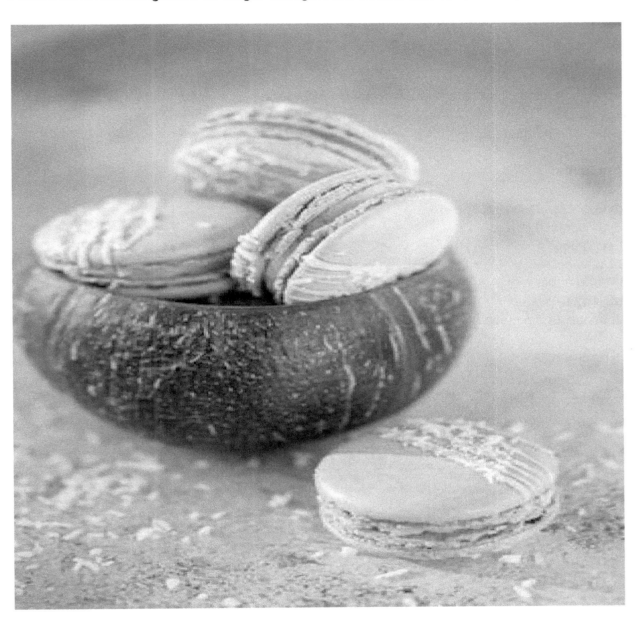

Chapter 7:

Beverages

7.1 Fresh Green Juice Blend

Fresh green juice blends are a fantastic way to incorporate a variety of nutrient-packed greens into your diet. This vibrant and refreshing juice combines different green vegetables for a boost of vitamins and minerals. Here's how to make it:

Ingredients:

- 2 cups kale leaves
- 1 cup spinach leaves
- 1 cucumber
- 2 stalks celery
- 1 green apple
- 1/2 lemon, peeled
- Optional: 1-inch piece of fresh ginger (for added flavor)

Instructions:

1. Wash all the vegetables and fruits thoroughly.

2. Cut the cucumber, celery, and green apple into smaller pieces that fit into your juicer.

3. Juice the kale, spinach, cucumber, celery, green apple, lemon, and ginger (if using) through a juicer according to its instructions. Make certain to squeeze out as much liquid as you can.

4. Once all the ingredients are juiced, give the mixture a good stir to combine the flavors.

5. Serve the fresh green juice immediately over ice or refrigerate for a short time before consuming to keep it cool.

6. Enjoy the refreshing and nutrient-rich green juice blend!

Note: You can customize this recipe by adding other greens such as Swiss chard, parsley, or romaine lettuce, according to your taste preferences. You can also adjust the sweetness and tartness by adding more or less green apple or lemon juice. Experiment with different combinations of greens to find your favorite blend. After using your juicer, don't forget to fully clean it.

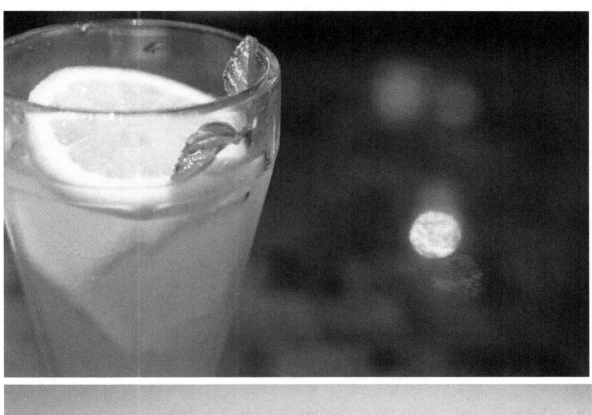

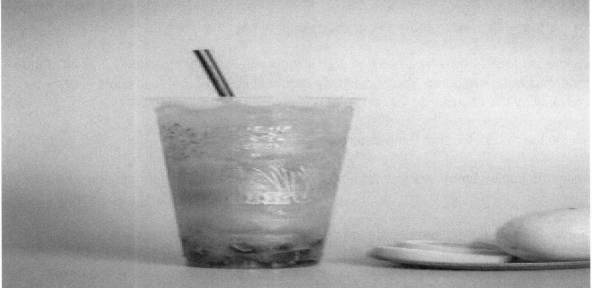

7.2 Homemade Iced Herbal Tea

Homemade iced herbal tea is a refreshing and hydrating beverage that can be customized with your favorite herbs and flavors. It's a perfect choice for hot summer days or whenever you need a cooling and flavorful drink. To get you started, here is a simple recipe:

Ingredients:

- 4 cups water
- 4 herbal tea bags or 4 tablespoons loose-leaf herbal tea
- Sweetener of choice (such as honey, maple syrup, or stevia) (optional)
- Sliced fruits, herbs, or citrus wedges for garnish (optional)
- Ice cubes

Instructions:

1. Heat the water in a kettle or saucepan to a rolling boil.

2. Remove the boiling water from the heat and add the herbal tea bags or loose-leaf herbal tea to the hot water. Steep according to the instructions provided for your specific herbal tea blend. Generally, herbal teas require steeping for 5-10 minutes.

3. Once the tea is steeped, remove the tea bags or strain out the loose tea leaves.

4. While the tea is still warm, sweeten it to your liking if you like. Stir thoroughly until all of the sweetener has been dissolved. You should be aware that some herbal teas could already be sweet or tasty by themselves, so you might not need any added sweetness.

5. Allow the tea to cool to room temperature.

6. Transfer the cooled herbal tea to a pitcher or glass jar and refrigerate for at least 1 hour to chill.

7. To serve, fill glasses with ice cubes and pour the chilled herbal tea over the ice.

8. If desired, garnish with sliced fruits, herbs, or citrus wedges for added flavor and visual appeal.

9. Stir the iced herbal tea before serving to distribute any settled flavors.

10. Enjoy your homemade iced herbal tea as a refreshing and soothing beverage!

Note: Feel free to experiment with different herbal tea blends and combinations to find your favorite flavors. You can also mix different herbs, such as mint or basil, to add a unique twist. Adjust the sweetness and garnishes according to your taste preferences. Leftover iced herbal tea can be stored in the refrigerator for a day or two, but it's best to consume it fresh for optimal taste and quality.

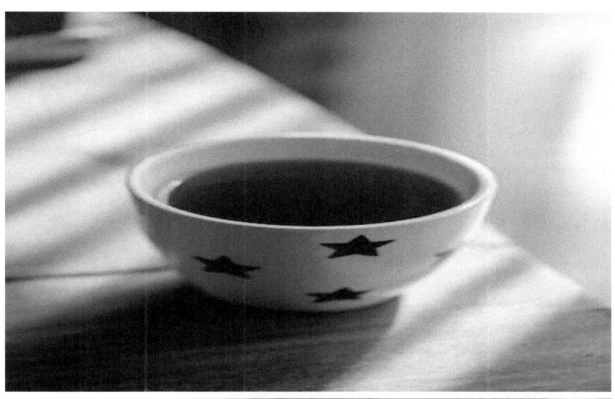

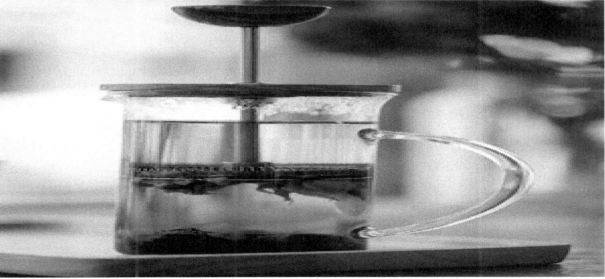

7.3 Detoxifying Infused Water

Detoxifying infused water is a hydrating and refreshing beverage that can help cleanse and rejuvenate your body. It's made by infusing water with a combination of fruits, vegetables, and herbs that are known for their detoxifying properties. To get you going, try this straightforward recipe:

Ingredients:

- 1 lemon, sliced
- 1 cucumber, sliced
- 10-12 fresh mint leaves
- 1-inch piece of fresh ginger, sliced (optional)
- 8 cups water

Instructions:

1. Wash the lemon, cucumber, mint leaves, and ginger (if using) thoroughly.

2. Slice the lemon and cucumber into thin rounds.

3. In a large pitcher, combine the lemon slices, cucumber slices, mint leaves, and ginger slices (if using).

4. Fill the pitcher with 8 cups of water.

5. Stir the ingredients gently to distribute the flavors.

6. Cover the pitcher and refrigerate for at least 2 hours, or preferably overnight, to allow the flavors to infuse into the water.

7. When you're ready to enjoy, give the infused water a gentle stir to enhance the flavors.

8. Pour the detoxifying infused water into glasses filled with ice cubes.

9. If desired, you can strain out the fruits and herbs before serving or leave them in the pitcher for a visually appealing presentation.

10. Sip on the detoxifying infused water throughout the day to stay hydrated and enjoy the cleansing benefits.

Note: You can customize this recipe by adding other detoxifying ingredients such as sliced strawberries, fresh basil, sliced oranges, or a pinch of cayenne pepper. Feel free to adjust the amount of each ingredient based on your taste preferences. You can refill the pitcher with water and continue to enjoy the infused flavors for up to 24 hours, but the fruits and herbs may start to lose their potency after that time. Remember to drink the infused water within a day or two for the best taste and freshness.

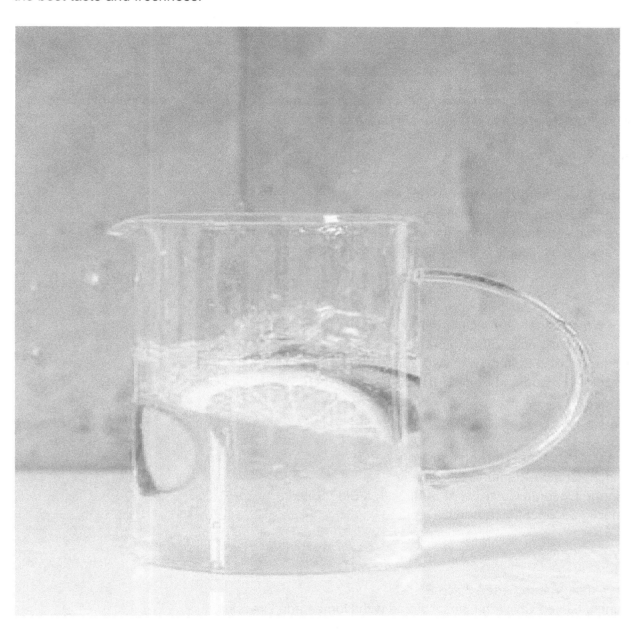

Chapter 8:

Meal Plans and Weekly Menus

8.1 One-Week Glucose Goddess Meal Plan

Sure! Here's a sample one-week Glucose Goddess meal plan to give you an idea of how to incorporate balanced and nutritious meals into your week:

Day 1:

- Breakfast: Energizing Morning Smoothie Bowl
- Lunch: Quinoa and Roasted Vegetable Salad
- Roasted vegetables and lemon-herb chicken on the grill for dinner
- Snack: Fresh Veggie Sticks with Greek Yogurt Dip

Day 2:

- Breakfast: Gluten-Free Quinoa Pancakes
- Lunch: Chickpea and Spinach Curry
- Dinner: Baked Salmon with Asparagus and Lemon-Dill Sauce
- Snack: Avocado and Black Bean Salsa with Whole Wheat Pita Chips

Day 3:

- Breakfast: Veggie-Packed Omelet
- Lunch: Quinoa-Stuffed Bell Peppers
- Dinner: Coconut Curry Lentil Soup with a Side Salad
- Snack: Coconut Macaroons

Day 4:

- Breakfast: Fresh Green Juice Blend
- Lunch: Grilled Chicken Caesar Salad with Homemade Dressing
- Dinner: Lemon-Herb Brown Rice Pilaf with Grilled Shrimp
- Snack: Raspberry Chia Seed Pudding

Day 5:

- Breakfast: Berry and Spinach Smoothie

- Lunch: Mediterranean Quinoa Salad
- Dinner: Garlic and Parmesan Roasted Brussels Sprouts with Grilled Steak
- Snack: Almond Butter Energy Balls

Day 6:

- Breakfast: Quinoa and Veggie Breakfast Burrito
- Lunch: Lentil and Vegetable Stir-Fry
- Dinner: Quinoa-Stuffed Zucchini Boats
- Snack: Whole Grain Crackers and Hummus with Carrot Sticks

Day 7:

- Breakfast: Overnight Chia Pudding with Fresh Fruit
- Lunch: Mixed Green Salad with Grilled Chicken, Avocado, and Balsamic Vinaigrette
- Dinner: Baked Cod with Lemon-Herb Sauce and Roasted Sweet Potato Fries
- Snack: Detoxifying Infused Water

Keep in mind to modify ingredients and portion amounts to suit your unique dietary requirements and tastes. Feel free to interchange meals between days or modify the recipes to suit your taste. It's also a good idea to consult with a healthcare professional or registered dietitian for personalized dietary advice. Enjoy your Glucose Goddess meal plan!

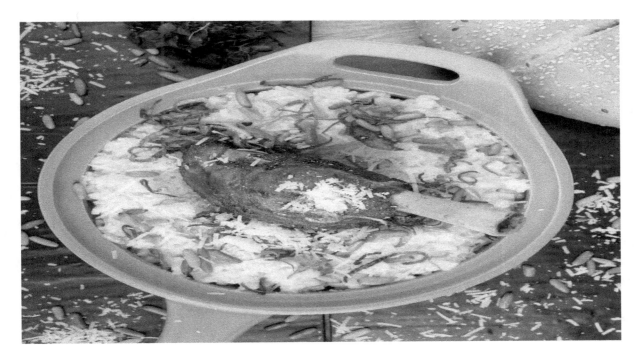

8.2 Grocery Shopping List for the Glucose Goddess Diet

Below is a grocery shopping list to help you get started with the Glucose Goddess Diet:

Proteins:
- Chicken breasts
- Salmon fillets
- Shrimp
- Eggs
- Greek yogurt
- Chickpeas
- Lentils

Vegetables:
- Kale
- Spinach
- Bell peppers
- Zucchini
- Eggplant
- Asparagus
- Brussels sprouts
- Sweet potatoes
- Onions
- Garlic
- Cucumber
- Celery
- Carrots
- Cherry tomatoes

Fruits:
- Berries (strawberries, raspberries, blueberries)
- Avocado
- Lemons
- Oranges
- Apples

Grains and Legumes:
- Quinoa
- Brown rice
- Whole wheat flour
- Gluten-free flour (if needed)
- Black beans

- Chia seeds

Dairy and Alternatives:
- Almond milk (unsweetened)
- Parmesan cheese (grated)
- Feta cheese (optional)
- Olive oil
- Coconut oil (optional)

Herbs and Spices:
- Fresh herbs (such as parsley, basil, dill, mint)
- Curry powder
- Ground cumin
- Ground coriander
- Turmeric
- Paprika
- Garlic powder
- Salt
- Pepper

Other Pantry Staples:
- Vegetable broth
- Balsamic vinegar
- Dijon mustard
- Maple syrup or honey (optional sweeteners)
- Almond butter
- Cocoa powder (if making desserts)

Snacks and Extras:
- Whole wheat pita chips
- Whole grain crackers
- Nuts (such as almonds)
- Seeds (such as sunflower seeds and chia seeds).
- Hummus
- Whole grain tortillas or wraps

It's important to note that this is a general shopping list, and you can adjust it based on your dietary preferences and needs. Consider any specific dietary restrictions or allergies you may have and customize the list accordingly. Don't forget to check your pantry for any items you may already have before heading to the store. Happy shopping and enjoy your Glucose Goddess Diet journey!

Chapter 9:

Guidelines for the Glucose Goddess Diet's Success

9.1 Mindful Eating and Portion Control

Mindful eating and portion control are essential practices to cultivate a healthy relationship with food and maintain a balanced diet. Here are some tips to help you practice mindful eating and portion control:

1. Eat slowly and savor each bite: Take the time to chew your food thoroughly and pay attention to the taste, texture, and flavors. Your body can detect fullness and satisfaction when you eat slowly.

2. Tune into your hunger and fullness cues: Before eating, assess your level of hunger on a scale from 1 to 10. Aim to eat when you are moderately hungry (around a 3-4) and stop eating when you are comfortably full (around a 6-7). Pay attention to your body's messages and obey them.

3. Use smaller plates and bowls: Serve your meals on smaller plates and bowls to help control portion sizes. Research has shown that people tend to eat less when using smaller dishware.

4. Pay attention to portion sizes: Familiarize yourself with recommended portion sizes for different food groups. Use measuring cups or a food scale to accurately portion out your meals, especially when starting out.

5. Include a variety of colors and textures: Aim to have a colorful plate by incorporating a variety of fruits, vegetables, whole grains, and lean proteins. This not only adds visual appeal but also provides a wide range of nutrients.

6. Be mindful of liquid calories: Beverages like sodas, juices, and sugary drinks can contribute to excess calorie intake. Opt for water, unsweetened herbal tea, or infused water as your main hydration sources.

7. Plan your meals and snacks: Plan your meals in advance and make a grocery list to ensure you have the necessary ingredients. You may make thoughtful decisions and avoid impulsive eating by keeping nutritious meals and snacks close at hand.

8. Practice portion control when dining out: Restaurants often serve larger portions, which can lead to overeating. Consider sharing a dish with a friend, ordering an appetizer-sized portion, or asking for a to-go box to save leftovers.

9. Focus on hunger and fullness, not external cues: Avoid eating solely based on external cues like the clock or emotions. Instead, check in with your body's hunger and fullness signals to guide your eating.

10. Be kind to yourself: Remember that mindful eating and portion control are ongoing practices. Embrace progress, not perfection, and approach your eating habits with self-compassion and understanding.

By incorporating these mindful eating and portion control strategies into your lifestyle, you can develop a healthier relationship with food, maintain a balanced diet, and support your overall well-being.

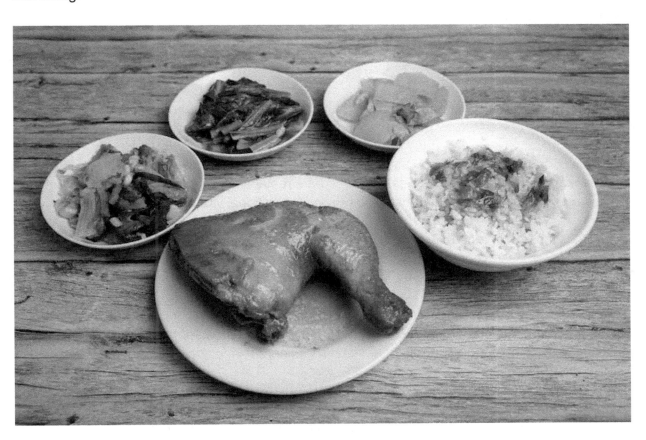

9.2 Smart Carbohydrate Swaps

Smart carbohydrate swaps are a great way to make healthier choices and incorporate nutrient-dense options into your diet. Here are some smart carbohydrate swaps to consider:

1. Whole grains instead of refined grains:
   - Choose whole wheat bread, whole grain pasta, and brown rice instead of their refined counterparts. More fiber, vitamins, and minerals are included in whole grains.

2. Sweet potatoes instead of white potatoes:
   - Sweet potatoes are packed with nutrients and have a lower glycemic index compared to white potatoes. They provide more fiber and vitamin A.

3. Quinoa instead of white rice:
   - Quinoa is a complete protein and contains more fiber than white rice. It is also rich in various minerals such as magnesium and iron.

4. Cauliflower rice instead of traditional rice:
   - Cauliflower rice is a low-carb alternative to rice that is high in fiber and rich in vitamins C and K. It can be easily prepared by pulsing cauliflower florets in a food processor.

5. Zucchini noodles instead of pasta:
   - Spiralized zucchini or "zoodles" can be used as a replacement for traditional pasta. Zucchini noodles are low in calories and carbs while providing additional vitamins and minerals.

6. Legumes instead of refined grains:
   - Include legumes in your meals, such as lentils, chickpeas, and black beans. They are high in fiber, protein, and beneficial nutrients.

7. Fresh fruits instead of processed snacks:
   - Choose fresh fruits for a natural source of carbohydrates instead of reaching for processed snacks high in refined sugars. Fruits offer vitamins, minerals, and fiber.

8. Whole grain crackers instead of regular crackers:
   - Opt for whole grain crackers made from whole wheat, oats, or other whole grains. They provide more fiber and nutrients compared to crackers made from refined flour.

9. Chia seeds instead of breadcrumbs:
   - Chia seeds can be used as a gluten-free alternative to breadcrumbs in recipes. They are rich in antioxidants, omega-3 fatty acids, and fiber.

10. Oatmeal instead of sugary cereals:

- Choose plain oats or steel-cut oats as a healthier alternative to sugary cereals. You can add flavor with fruits, nuts, or a touch of honey or cinnamon.

These smart carbohydrate swaps allow you to maintain a balanced diet while incorporating more nutrient-dense options. Remember to consider portion sizes and listen to your body's hunger and fullness cues. Consult a qualified dietician or healthcare provider for customized recommendations based on your unique dietary requirements and health goals.

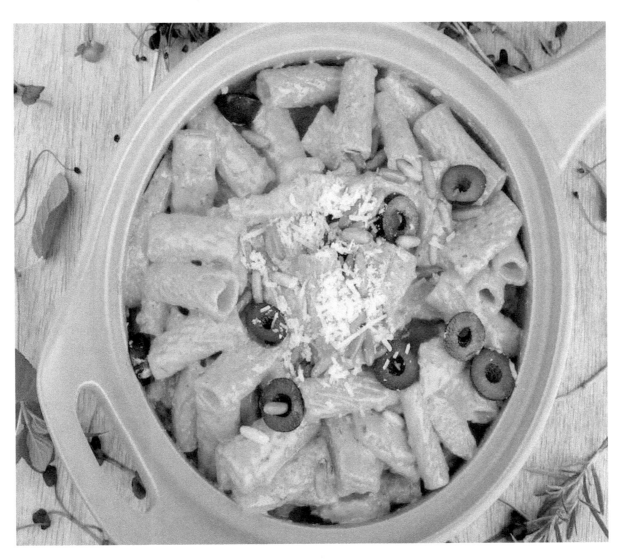

9.3 Dining Out and Traveling on the Glucose Goddess Diet

Dining out and traveling while following the Glucose Goddess Diet may require some extra planning and mindful choices. Here are some tips to help you navigate dining out and traveling while sticking to your dietary goals:

1. Research restaurants and menu options: Before dining out, take some time to research restaurants in the area and review their menus online. Look for options that align with the Glucose Goddess Diet, such as those offering lean proteins, vegetables, whole grains, and healthier cooking methods.

2. Make special requests: Don't hesitate to make special requests when ordering your meal. Ask for dressings or sauces on the side, request steamed or grilled preparations instead of fried, and substitute sides for healthier options like steamed vegetables or a side salad.

3. Opt for protein and vegetable-based dishes: Choose dishes that feature lean proteins like grilled chicken, fish, or tofu, along with a generous serving of vegetables. This helps to ensure a balanced meal with a focus on nutrient-dense ingredients.

4. Portion control: Be mindful of portion sizes, as restaurants often serve larger portions. Consider sharing a meal with a friend or packing up leftovers to enjoy later.

5. Be cautious with condiments and sauces: Many sauces and dressings can be high in added sugars or unhealthy fats. Ask for sauces and dressings on the side, and use them sparingly or opt for healthier alternatives like olive oil, vinegar, or lemon juice.

6. Stay hydrated: It's important to stay hydrated while traveling. To make sure you have access to water all day, keep a reusable water bottle with you. Avoid sugary drinks and opt for unsweetened herbal tea or infused water when available.

7. Pack healthy snacks: When traveling, bring along healthy snacks to have on hand. This helps you avoid relying on unhealthy options during transit or when faced with limited food choices. Pack nuts, seeds, cut-up vegetables, or homemade energy bars to keep you fueled.

8. Plan ahead: If possible, plan your meals in advance. Look for grocery stores or markets at your travel destination to purchase fresh fruits, vegetables, and other Glucose Goddess Diet-friendly ingredients. This allows you to have control over your meals and make healthier choices.

9. Practice moderation: While it's important to maintain your dietary goals, remember that occasional indulgences are part of a balanced lifestyle. Allow yourself to enjoy a treat or try local cuisine in moderation, while still making mindful choices overall.

10. Listen to your body: Pay attention to your body's hunger and fullness cues. Eat when you're hungry and stop when you're satisfied. Practice mindful eating and be present with your meals, enjoying the flavors and textures.

Remember that flexibility and adaptation are key when dining out and traveling. Prioritize making the best choices available to you, while also being kind to yourself and enjoying your experiences.

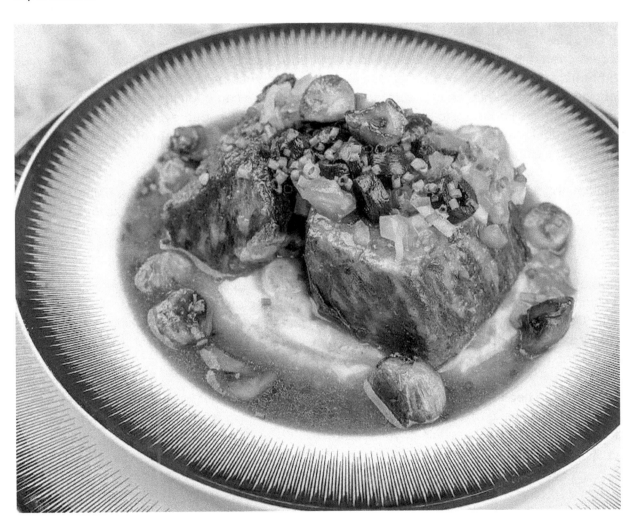

Chapter 10:

Conclusion:

Embracing a Healthier, Balanced Lifestyle

Embracing a healthier, balanced lifestyle is a wonderful choice for your overall well-being. By incorporating the principles of the Glucose Goddess Diet, such as focusing on whole foods, balancing macronutrients, and practicing portion control, you can nourish your body and support optimal health. It's important to remember that healthy eating is a journey, and it's okay to have occasional indulgences and setbacks along the way. The key is to cultivate mindfulness, listen to your body's signals, and make choices that align with your health goals.

In addition to following a nutritious diet, remember to prioritize other aspects of a balanced lifestyle. Engage in regular physical activity, prioritize quality sleep, manage stress levels, and foster healthy relationships. As vital as looking after your physical health is looking after your mental and emotional wellbeing.

As you continue on your journey towards a healthier, balanced lifestyle, remember to be patient and kind to yourself. It's normal to encounter challenges and setbacks, but every step forward counts. Celebrate your progress and focus on the positive changes you're making in your life. Consider seeking support from a healthcare professional or registered dietitian who can provide personalized guidance and help you stay on track.

By embracing a healthier, balanced lifestyle, you're investing in your long-term health and well-being. Enjoy the journey and the positive impact it will have on your life. You deserve to feel your best and thrive in all aspects of your being.

www.ingramcontent.com/pod-product-compliance
Lightning Source LLC
LaVergne TN
LVHW081817161224
799261LV00042B/869